The Gay Men's Guide to Glory Holes

What Every Man—Gay or Straight—Needs to Know About Glory Holes

PUBLISHED BY: Bathhouse Blues

ISBN: 9798224151608

I've tried to recreate events, locales, and conversations from my memories. In some instances, I changed the names of individuals and places to maintain their anonymity; I may have changed some identifying characteristics and details, such as physical properties, occupations, and places of residence.

DISCLAIMER

The material in this book is for adults only. The First Amendment of the United States of America Constitution and the Canadian Charter of Rights and Freedoms protect this book as a reference work for educational, informational, archival, entertainment, and other purposes.

This book offers no medical, legal, or related professional advice. We encourage the reader to apply the contained information with sound judgment and seek advice from a qualified professional when necessary. At best, the content provided in this book is of a general nature. The purpose of this book is to enhance, not replace, intimate relationships with another individual.

This text should not be considered advice for illegal activities. This text is for private consumption only. By using any of the material in this book, you agree that you know your local laws and accept 100% personal liability for any illegal actions you commit.

The author advocates absolutely no illegal activities of any kind and makes no express or implied warranties of merchantability, fitness for any purpose, or otherwise concerning this book, all references, and the information it contains. The author urges you to consult the appropriate licensed practitioner for medical, legal, or spiritual advice.

Neither the publisher nor the author shall be liable for any commercial damages, including but not limited to special, incidental, consequential, or other damages.

Before engaging in any sexual activity, be sure that you do not take risks beyond your level of experience, aptitude, and comfort.

Meeting someone online is overwhelmingly safe. Most people you meet online are truthful and well-founded.

Nothing is ever 100% safe. For your protection, always keep a record of where you are going and send the information to a friend. Never give your home phone number to a stranger. Always assume the person you are hooking up with is HIV positive.

Please do not take for granted that your partner will protect himself. It is your responsibility to play safe. People from all over the world are meeting in person and making their first contact online. These meetings result in very few violent crimes.

In the world of glory holes, poppers are the most common. Know beforehand how Amyl Nitrite might affect you both physically and mentally. In addition, research indicates mixing more than one party drug in the equation often leads to unsafe sex.

MORE TITLES BY THIS AUTHOR

Bathhouse Blues
Your Guide to Gay Bathhouses

No Asians Please
How Asian Men Are Perceived in The Gay Community

Gay Steam
True Sex Tales from The Tubs

Back To the Baths
More Gay Bathhouse Stories

DEDICATION
To Danny Z. - Thanks for The Free Hosting.

TABLE OF CONTENTS

INTRODUCTION

Who would have thought that a pandemic would make Glory Holes mainstream? Cities under lockdown experienced exactly that. In the beginning, places like the New York City Health Department told its residents that they should look to alternative methods if they needed to be sexually active. "Physical barriers, such as walls, facilitate sexual interaction while hindering intimate face-to-face interaction."

Naturally, many people seized upon this information—the New York City Health Department was promoting the use of Glory Holes.
One province in Canada took an initiative-taking approach. British Columbia put out a pamphlet encouraging its use, complete with instructions on how one uses a Glory Hole.

No one has ever authored a comprehensive book about Glory Hole culture and its unwritten rules. It is ironic since Glory Holes have endured for decades.

So why author a book about Glory Holes? For the same reason, I authored a book about bathhouses. On the web, you can find plenty of erotic stories about Glory Holes. But just like the baths, not much is written about them, etiquette-wise. These avenues for anonymous sex have been widespread but rarely discussed. That is, until now.

There are thousands of men, both straight and gay, who are curious about the Glory Hole world. But they are too scared to give it a shot. Since this is a book for gay men, the material will focus exclusively on the gay male perspective—spanning from its evolution as a sex culture to its unspoken etiquette rules.

In contrast to my knowledge of gay baths, I am not an expert when it comes to Glory Holes. All I have been able to do is write down my observations of Glory Hole action at the baths. Cruising for sex at the baths is like cruising for sex around Glory Holes. While there is hardly any eye contact, the moves and signals are quite similar.

So, what is the bottom line? Glory Holes truly represent what quick, dark, anonymous, depersonalized sex is all about.

CHAPTER 1
The Five Ws
What is a Glory Hole?

Picture two people situated face-to-face with a wall between them. Imagine the same wall, but with a hole located directly around the person's genital area. One person sticks out their cock, and the other sucks it off. Is the concept that simple? It is.

Glory Holes have been around for centuries. But for this book, I will focus on recent times, beginning in the 1950s. Ironically, it was bi-curious guys who started boosting the underground popularity of Glory Holes. Back then, sex was considered taboo, a subject you never talked about.

Many women from that era viewed sex as a function of either procreation or fulfilling their wifely duties. Most wives would only participate in intercourse. However, during that period, oral sex was considered impure despite men's desire for more. These men had no choice but to seek oral sex elsewhere. Both then and now, Glory Holes provide complete anonymity, with only a hole in the wall. Neither party would know who is behind the hole. Guaranteeing complete secrecy. Privacy was necessary, as it would be scandalous for anyone to find out that a guy (especially if married) was engaging in man-on-man sex. Word of mouth was the only way to find a place for a glory hole.

The 60s and 70s brought the concept of Glory Holes into the adult bookstores, with women entering the fray as the givers (more on that later). However, you would also find queer adult bookstores, where gay and closeted men would cruise the stalls to either give or receive.

Though the AIDS crisis hit the eighties hard, Glory Holes were still in demand because oral sex was (and still is) a low-risk activity for HIV infection. However, oral sex can transmit other STIs (sexually transmitted infections). Later in this book, we will delve deeper into that topic.

Today, Glory Holes seem to be everywhere, and their popularity has not slowed down. Its notoriety has even bled into the mainstream, appearing in such films as Scary Movie. However, Glory Holes remain so hidden from the general public that many people still struggle to locate them. Why does it have such enduring appeal? One reason is that the concept is relatively simple: a hole in the wall. When one shuts down, ten others can easily appear somewhere else.

You can find them in large urban centers, remote rural areas, adult bookstores, public restrooms, gay video booths, and even people's homes. With the advent of the Internet, it is much easier to advertise. Numerous discussion boards exist for users to express their opinions about various Glory Holes and their locations. However, one must exercise extreme caution, as public sex remains illegal. Even as a consenting adult, the police could still arrest you for lewd conduct. Just ask George Michael.

Why Do Guys Go?

Bottom line: guys want to get off. They do not want an intimate bonding experience. Men prefer their interactions to be swift and direct. They are not interested in introductions, getting to know you, or exchanging numbers. They want that satisfaction without any strings attached. However, some guys enjoy the thrill of the chase, the unspoken moves, and the cruising.

In some cases, the risk of getting caught in public is such a thrill—a high that no drug can manufacture. Its existence also enables men to rationalize their actions as a means of simply getting off. straight and married guys do not see this activity as cheating. For these men, oral sex is not "sex," as there was no intercourse. What should they do if their spouse will not give them oral sex? That is where the Glory Holes come in.

But why seek out Glory Holes? You cut right to the chase, as that cock is hanging out of a glory hole waiting to be sucked. There is no need to play endless games or waste time searching for a cock online or in bars. You would think Glory Hole locations would become obsolete with the advent of online cruising for sex. But the opposite is true. Guys seeking sexual pleasure continue to frequent these places. Instead of spending money on a date with no guarantee of getting anything, it is cheaper to cruise for action at the Glory Holes.

You would think that oral sex would be a personal, intimate, bonding experience between two people who genuinely care for one another. It is an opportunity to let go and give completely to the other person. However, break free from a heterosexual perspective. In the gay community, the opposite is true. Kissing is the equivalent of displaying intimate contact between two guys who genuinely love each other. Being blown or laid is something you can experience anywhere. Gay men prefer to reserve actual, physical, intimate contact, such as kissing, for their future boyfriends. Many men have confided in me that they refrain from kissing other men with whom they are involved. Oral sex? No problem. Anal? Pass the lube. But kissing? NO WAY! You would anticipate the opposite to be true.

But there is also an underlying element to all of this. Casual sex is all about connecting with someone else. Many guys are just so damn lonely that they need an outlet. Oral sex is all about forging that connection with another person, however fleeting.

Making a short-term connection is the bottom line. These men are not looking for a relationship or even a friendship. Therefore, if your goal is to find a relationship, do not expect to find one while cruising Glory Holes. These sessions last 5 to 10 minutes, tops, if you are lucky. Additionally, many of these guys snort poppers to achieve an extra high. Once someone unloads, it is over. That is, until someone new starts lurking around the Glory Hole looking for action.

Who Are the Guys That Go?

Mention the term "Glory Holes," and people perceive them as a haven of uncleanliness, isolated in a shaded setting. People often assume glory holes only attract sex addicts, drug users, and dirty older men dressed in raincoats. Yes, there are people like that. However, there is also a broad cross-section of men who frequent these holes. The crowd is ethnically diverse, consisting of Black men, Asians, Twinks, muscular hunks, and others. They range from husbands who cannot get oral sex from their wives to gay men who love the thrill of cruising. All these men have one thing in common. They want cock.

There are some men do not give much thought to attaching a face to the cock they are sucking. A cock is just a cock. However, most guys tend to be selective about which dick they choose to suck. The urge to put a face on the cock is prevalent. Several men peek through the hole, and if the guy is not their type, they take a pass. This undermines the essence of what a glory hole symbolizes: endlessly sucking off cocks with complete abandonment. However, most men need to have a mental image of the guy in their minds before they initiate oral sex, so expect rejection. Sad but true.

When Do Guys Go?

You will find a variety of different guys ready to play. Your experience will vary depending on the time you visit the Glory Holes. During the day, you will encounter men squeezing in that quickie before work, between appointments, or on their way home. On the other hand, you will come across men who stop by after a date in the evenings because they could not get to second base. So, they swing by for a quick cock suck. Go in, blow, and then go. It is so quick and easy.

In the late hours of the night, you will encounter a multitude of guys who have exhausted their options at the bars and clubs. Meanwhile, there are others who are heavily intoxicated or under the influence. However, they have not experienced any sexual encounters, making this their final option before ending the night. Between those times, you will find men spending time together at the glory holes who enjoy chasing and cruising all those cocks.

CHAPTER 2
Where Can You Find A Glory Hole?

The internet has made it much easier to find a hole. In the olden days, you had to rely on word of mouth. If that did not work, you could find listings of Glory Holes in the classified sections on the back pages of gay magazines.

Nowadays, with just a click of the mouse, you can find many places with a Glory Hole. While it may not be as comprehensive as the Yellow Pages, it is still a valuable resource. With Internet cruising, you can break it into three categories: discussion boards, online classifieds, and hookup sites. Only individuals aged 18 and above can access these three online venues.

It is **your responsibility** to make sure whomever you are hooking up with is a consenting adult.

Online Classified

Craigslist used to be the best place to post an adult classified ad. This was the case until Craigslist discontinued their listings for adult services. However, many free online classified forums allow you to post ads. However, if you google for "Craigslist Killer," a variety of dangers and risks will appear on your screen. In a public bathroom, looking for Glory Hole action is dangerous. The individuals who respond to your ad could range from homophobic individuals to law enforcement officer's eager to conduct a raid. Realistically, it is doubtful that the police have the time or the resources to scan online postings to make a bust. But you also cannot rule it out.

Posting online also exposes you to potential harassment from psychos or gay bashers who are seeking to cause you harm. Your best bet in placing ads is meeting at venues in a controlled environment. If you place an ad saying you are looking for Glory Hole action in either a bathhouse or sex club, it is doubtful any gay-basher or psycho will show up.

These establishments provide a sexualized gay environment, which may be outside their comfort zone.

Then there is the "At Home" Glory Holes. This refers to instances where men have established a glory hole within their own homes. Those who host the Glory Hole are more at risk than visitors. We will discuss the risks associated with hosting the Glory Hole later in this book, as the host has no idea who will show up.

However, anyone arranging a hookup would encounter issues like these. Hosting requires a decision to accept those risks. Otherwise, there are other venues you can choose to meet up at, like a bookstore, bathhouse, sex club, etc.

If you still insist on going this way, get the person's email address. To see what comes up, Google their handle and email. If many gay-related profiles appear, then the person is probably legit. If no profiles appear, exercise caution and consider passing on hooking up with this person. If you decide to go ahead and become a victim of assault and robbery, you will still have their email information. Plus, your ISP will be recording the person's IP address. So at least the police officers have a starting point to find the person. But this would be an extreme case. However, it is advisable to prioritize safety over regret in the long term.

Discussion Boards

If you want to get more involved in Glory Holes, it is best to communicate with other like-minded people who engage in this activity. For those who are new to the scene, it serves as an excellent opportunity to acquaint themselves, from seeking advice to receiving pointers from more experienced individuals. You can learn a tremendous amount from what others post on discussion boards. Here are a few of the best places to get involved and start chatting with others about the topic. These are sites that exclusively cater to the gay community.

gloryholeguide.com

The Glory Hole Guide allows you to discuss etiquette, fantasies, and encounters. It features the latest Glory Hole locations, videos, pictures, and erotic stories. Discussion threads also allow newcomers to interact online with the Gay Glory Hole community.

squirt.org

While Squirt is primarily known for its cruising and hookups, it offers a unique feature that no other website can match. Squirt provides regular updates on over 15,000 public locations worldwide where gay men can meet for sex. Locations include local parks, change areas, public toilets, bars, sex clubs, and bathhouses.

Every listing describes the characteristics of each location. Each venue's discussion boards allow users to post questions and interact with other users. Since this is a global platform, you can also explore other locations. Therefore, if you are a frequent traveler, you can explore the nearby Glory Hole locations. You can post questions and interact with those local users.

address4sex.com

I'm not familiar with this website, so I can only describe what I've seen. It features listings for gay, straight, and bi men who search for sex at local cruising places. One aspect that sets this site apart from Squirt.org is its emphasis on Glory Holes. The search function allows users to type in their postal/zip code and locate Glory Holes nearby. Users can also place ads and interact with other members interested in Glory Hole action.

lpsg.com

For those fascinated with cock, LPSG stands for Long Penis Support Group. Its audience is a vast community of people who identify as straight, gay, and bi-curious. By signing up, you can search out past posts about Glory Holes. This feature enables users to thoroughly research and identify the top cruise destinations. You can also ask and receive feedback by posting questions and queries. You might even start conversing with other posters and arrange a hookup.

Hookup Sites

Most of the hookup sites are not Glory Hole friendly, as guys are looking for one-on-one action at someone's place. But not all is lost. There are a few hookup sites that offer Glory Hole action. The following sites cater exclusively to the gay community.

gloryhole.directory

Glory Holes now have a new global directory. Those who create a Glory Hole must sign up and create a free listing. This site supports and promotes Glory Holes all over the world.

cumhunt.com

Cumhunt is a dating site for those who are only interested in oral sex—giving, receiving, and cum eating. Since sucking and Glory Holes go hand in hand, this would be a fantastic place to find guys who might also be interested in this type of action. You can also engage in chats with guys, send video messages, and maintain a list of your favorite cock suckers.

gloryshole.com

Here, you will find a directory of locations worldwide, along with a map of places and spots featuring Glory Holes.

truckersucker.com

Trucker sucker is precisely as its name suggests—truckers looking to suck. That is all. This is not a place for a date, a relationship, or even a long-term one-night stand. These truckers want a blowjob, period. So, post your profile and start searching for truckers passing by your town.

recon.com

Recon is the go-to place if you want to find someone with any fetish. Many of its members have their own 'chamber,' including an at-home Glory Hole. It would be presumptuous to assume that the site's thousands of members are exclusively interested in Glory Holes. It will take a lot of weeding out of profiles to narrow down your search for that Glory Hole guy. With a little assistance from this website, you can do it!

reddit.com/r/GloryHoleLocations/

This section on Reddit resembles Craigslist before they (Craigslist) discontinued their adult postings. This page serves as a central location for people to list the private glory holes they are hosting. Additionally, this page posts listings for public Glory Hole locations. These locations range from cruising spots, public play areas, and hookup spots on college campuses, among others.

Apps

It's surprising that there isn't an app for locating nearby Glory Holes, given the prevalence of apps for almost everything. Well, that is not true. There is a Glory Hole app, but it primarily caters to the heterosexual community. Therefore, you will only encounter women.

You could seek out Glory Hole action using the hookup app you personally use; Grindr is a perfect example. I'd prefer not to recommend a particular gay hookup app, as so many exist. However, expect a low response rate for Glory Hole hookups. These apps seem to be much more superficial in what men are seeking. Guys want to see both the body and the face—no pic, no response.

Most of the gay men on these apps are out and proud. They prefer one-on-one anal sex with a hot man, as opposed to anonymous oral sex through a hole. The harsh truth is that most men seek a hookup that includes anal, oral, rimming, and kissing. That is the reality. Until developers develop an app specifically for gay glory hole action, searching for an anonymous blow job on a hookup app is like trying to find a needle in a haystack.

CHAPTER 3
Glory Hole Etiquette

One rule for both the giver and receiver: always carry TONS of Kleenex or paper napkins with you. It is essential for both the giver and receiver to carry tons of tissues. You can never predict the extent of the release. It could be a squirt, or it could be a river of ejaculate. No matter what happens, the end will be sticky. It is wise to clean up the mess afterward.

Receiving

Before you stick your cock through the hole, look at the hole itself. Are there sharp edges around the hole? Does the hole look clean? Is the hole large enough to force your entire body against it? Before starting, it would be beneficial to consider these factors to prevent any potential injuries.

After examining the hole, you are now ready for Glory Hole action. If you don't care who does the oral, stick your cock through and wait for the parade of mouths to start sucking. If you are like most men, you are selective about who you allow to perform oral sex on you. Here's how to identify and screen those who are not worthy of your trust.

Don't stick your cock immediately through the hole. Peek through and see who is lurking on the other side. If there is someone you like, try to get the sucker's attention. Draw a circle around the interior of the glory hole itself. You're expressing your direct desire for a blowjob. But what if you find the person unattractive? Don't stick your cock through the hole. It is that simple. The giver may open his mouth wide against the hole, indicating that he wants to suck you off. If you have no interest, don't respond. Just stand there and wait until he leaves. He will eventually understand the hint. However, if he is persistent and won't leave, cover the hole with your hand. This is a clear indication that you have no desire for him. That is a more hurtful sign, but sometimes you need to be brutal to get your point across. This type of cruising is not for the timid, as rejection is a common occurrence. If you find this unacceptable, pursuing glory hole sex is not for you.

Above all, keep standing straight. Depending on where you go for Glory Hole action, there might be hours and hours of standing and waiting for that blowjob. It is essential to maintain proper posture, as you want to avoid wearing out your spine.

Giving

The allure of Glory Holes lies in their abundance of riches, as they offer a buyers' market of cocks. Glory Holes are ideal for those who enjoy constant suckling and don't care about the origin of the cock. However, many men who identify as givers are just as selective as the receivers I write about. Not only do they gravitate towards the head of the cock, but also towards the head resting on those shoulders.

However, you should also enjoy the act of oral sex. Think about quality, not quantity. Take your time and savor the experience. Slow down and try to be tender and non-aggressive. This approach is far more effective than attempting to suck as many people as possible in an hour.

Some tips: Don't begin by jacking off that cock with your hands. That tends to kill the mood. Glory Holes are sucking, not jerking off their cocks; if the receiver wants a handjob, he can do it himself.

Avoid biting down and using your teeth. You're sucking the cock, not eating it. Using teeth is just improper etiquette and unacceptable manners.

You'll be able to tell when the other person is ready to end the sucking session. While you may want to continue, the other person may not feel the same way. There can be many reasons why the person doesn't want to go on. If the guy doesn't want to ejaculate, it's not your fault. Don't press the issue because you will appear clingy. Accept the end of the sucking session gracefully and move on to the next person.

Avoid brushing your teeth before you engage in oral sex. Additionally, refrain from eating a meal prior to engaging in oral sex. Both activities irritate your gums, which may increase your chances of catching an STI. If you are worried about your breath, pop a mint. Don't chew but let the mint sit on your tongue and dissolve.

Gestures and Their Meaning

Hand gestures around the hole (by the receiver).

- Signal that he wants you to suck his cock.

Face in front of the Glory Hole.

- He wants to suck your cock, NOW.

Either the giver or the receiver obstructs the hole.

- The individual has no interest in getting sucked or sucking someone else.

Either party (giver or receiver) starts to seem disinterested.

- This indicates that he has had enough and wants to move on.

Sucking Gets Terminated quickly and abruptly. Some scenarios could have occurred:

- The guy receiving a blowjob finds it painful. Maybe the sucker used his teeth, went down too deep, or felt too sharp. Regardless of the situation, the guy finds it too painful to endure the sucking.

- Alternatively, the man is on the verge of exploding and is reluctant to ejaculate at this moment, especially if he wishes to attract multiple men.

Ejaculating In the Mouth Of A Guy

Despite being in an enclosed space, Glory Holes lacks soundproofing. On the other side, someone can hear you. If you are about to ejaculate, it is responsible etiquette to say, "I'm going to cum." Seriously, it is that simple. Informing the recipient would be beneficial.

It is up to the receiving person to warn that ejaculation is imminent. However, men who typically receive do not climax. Why is that? This is due to the significant decrease in sex drive that occurs after ejaculation. These guys want as much oral sex as possible. So, they hold back. Otherwise, why bother hanging around?

This doesn't bode well for some givers who aim to consume multiple streams of warm cum. This is why some individuals strive to suck as many cocks as possible. They understand that eventually they will achieve success and experience an explosion in their mouths. Although oral sex poses a low risk for HIV infection, it does not eliminate the possibility of contracting a different STI. Using mouthwash after every sucking experience only helps slightly; it is not considered a tool for STI prevention. But it doesn't hurt to take all possible precautions.

Some guys give no warning whatsoever when they are about to ejaculate. They just explode. Sometimes it is accidental, as they are so caught up in the moment that they don't realize they've climaxed. Others don't care. You are merely a mouthpiece, so what does it matter? But most times, you can tell.

Again, the walls are not soundproof. When a guy is about to cum, they will let you know. Heavy breathing, gasps, grunts, and exclamations of "I'm about to cum" are some indicators. If you prefer not to have ejaculate in your mouth, withdraw and provide him with a hand job until he ejaculates. If he asks why you stopped, say you don't swallow.

What would happen if the situation escalated to the point where he ejaculated directly into your mouth? Immediately swallow it or spit it out. This underscores the importance of always carrying Kleenex. Yes, oral sex is a low-risk activity, but that doesn't mean there is no risk. Ensure that your annual physicals include STI testing. If you have no primary care doctor, try to find a local gay men's health clinic that provides STI testing. Regardless of whether a man has ejaculated in your mouth or not, you should undergo this type of testing at least once a year.

Dos & Don'ts

Show consideration for your partner.

It would be disrespectful to deny the giver a protein shot if he asks for it. Don't hold anything back; if he requests it, unload it on the sucking guy.

Make sure your cock is clean.

Don't hang around in a booth if you are not using it. You deny space to someone else.

Rock-hard cocks are necessary to achieve a blowjob. Limp won't cut it. Either take Viagra or wear a cock ring.

If one guy is serving many others in a row, don't cut in front of the line. Be patient and wait for your turn.

If you are not interested in getting sucked by someone, be clear and say no. Don't lead someone on. You are both wasting time.

Shyness doesn't work. If you can't manage to be upfront and direct about sucking or being sucked, stay away from these places.

Glory Holes are not a social setting; this is simply anonymous sex. Keep chitchat to a minimum. Some conversations do happen, but not often. Guys are there to engage in oral sex—neither more nor less.

Avoid putting your hand through the hole and grabbing someone. Circle your finger around the hole to show interest.

Shove your cock through the hole to show it off to shoppers looking to suck.

If you want to piss in the guy's mouth, ask first.

Dirty talk is okay, as is moaning and groaning with pleasure.

Don't ask for phone numbers or email addresses. Most guys aren't there to find friends or partners. They're there for oral sex, period.

Anal Sex

Let me preface this by saying that other than a monogamous relationship, I don't support or encourage bareback sex in any situation. But at the same time, who am I to judge someone else's behavior? What works for you might not work for me, and vice versa. Who am I to tell you what to do? We all have choices. I may not choose unsafe sex, but I cannot choose for you.

This book would not be complete without discussing fucking or getting fucked through a glory hole. 99% of the anal sex that takes place is bareback. If you find the concept uncomfortable, proceed to the next section of this chapter. If you practice bareback sex in your private life and have no problem with it, start reading below. However, keep in mind that every cock that touches your butt might have touched 20 other butts before yours. And it's only been an hour. Therefore, always prepare ahead of time to ensure your ass is clean and tidy, so douche.

Let's put the moralizing aside and talk about where to find anal sex in a Glory Hole setting. If you are a top, it's going to be a challenging endeavor. Oral sex is the primary use of glory holes. So, it will be challenging to find someone who is willing to fuck through a hole. But it's not entirely impossible. People often believe that the tops hold all the power in any encounter. Adding glory holes to the equation reveals that the power lies with the bottom. How? Tops cannot fuck until bottoms arrive on the scene.

As a top, you are at the mercy of the bottoms. You can't do anything until the bottoms arrive on site. You need to wait it out. The sole drawback of the bottom is that it is necessary to suck multiple men to find one who is interested in fucking your ass. To find someone like that, you must first assume the role of the giver. Here is how to do it. Crouch in front of the hole and wait for someone to arrive. When they do, circle the hole with your finger to indicate your interest. When a cock appears through the Glory Hole, start sucking. After a period, remove your mouth and begin to stroke the man's genitalia with your hand while standing. Next, rotate your body to face the erect cock and continue to stroke it. Finally, insert the cock into your ass and start pumping. It feels like having sex while squatting, but you're in a bizarre position. It reads more manageable than it sounds, but you need experience to successfully pull it off.

Practice at home a few times, placing a dildo on the wall to make the transition as smooth as possible. However, keep in mind that this is a Glory Hole. Guys are looking for oral, not anal. Therefore, anticipate frequent rejection. Not all guys will engage in fucking through a hole. Some guys will stop and leave because they don't want to engage in anal, especially without a condom. But some guys will go for it. They are either caught up in the moment or searching for a bottom. Only when the stars and moon align perfectly can anal sex occur, making it unpredictable. The guys you encounter at the Glory Holes are more into sucking than fucking. Expect a significant number of guys to walk away. However, finding a Glory Hole top is not impossible. It just takes a lot of patience and waiting.

CHAPTER 4
STI, Safety, Legalities
STI

I argue that the same concerns about the spread of STIs (sexually transmitted infections) at the gay baths also apply to Glory Hole locations. It's not the location of sexual activity that spreads sexually transmitted infections—it's the individual engaging in it. The only safe sex is no sex. If that's not possible, safer sex is your only option. You could meet a guy online and go back to his place. At the baths, you could hook up with someone. You could even contract a sexually transmitted infection (STI) from a partner who has cheated. The point is, sexually transmitted infections (STIs) do not choose a specific venue to spread; rather, it is the individual. So, we all need to take responsibility for our own behavior, as actions have consequences.

If you are a married or closeted man with a partner who believes that condom use is the most effective form of protection during oral sex, **STOP RIGHT HERE**. Sucking or getting sucked while wearing a condom will never happen. I can't speak for women when it comes to Glory Hole sex. Gay men will not use a condom during oral sex. Period. They want the taste of cock on their lips and mouths. This also applies to gay men who desire the sensation of another man's tongue slurping their dick. The bottom line is that a cock in a condom will be rejected, as gay men do not suck cock using a condom.

While the risk is relatively low for an STI transmission, there is still risk. Regular STI checks are the norm for most gay men. Therefore, even if they catch something, medication can often clear it up. This is not the case for married men or heterosexual individuals in a committed relationship. How can you persuade your significant other to undergo an STI test if you are supposedly monogamous? What if your result comes back positive? What do you do? Leaving an STI untreated could result in fatal consequences for the unsuspecting partner.

The positive news for guys who are only interested in receiving oral sex is that the risk of contracting a sexually transmitted infection (STI) is extremely low, potentially zero. However, if you engage in regular cocksucking, it's advisable to undergo testing. Aim for a test at least once a year, just for your peace of mind. What if you're married and suck cock on the side? There are many STIs you can get from oral sex. Even if the man doesn't ejaculate in your mouth, the risk remains. Even though the risk decreases, we cannot rule out pre-cum as a factor.

Only you will be able to decide how to move forward. Is your desire for oral sex such that you're willing to disrupt your current relationship? Even if the risk is small? At that point, you should seek advice from a specialist in STIs. They would know best how to advise you.

If you decide to go this route, choose only ONE STI specialist to talk to. Not all STI specialists think the same way. While they have similar roadmaps to follow, each has their own opinion. Consulting various experts will make all that advice spin in your head. Every piece of advice contradicts the next, confusing you more. Pick one specialist, stick with it, and move forward. Though this specialist will give you the best advice, only you can decide how far you want to go.

Let's talk about the drug use that occurs at these Glory Holes. Poppers are most prevalent in the world of oral sex. Know beforehand how Amyl Nitrite might affect you both physically and mentally. Also, research how mixing more than one party drug can often lead to unsafe sex. So, keep that in mind.

Safety

I briefly discussed safety in the section about online classifieds. I address the remaining concerns regarding one's safety in this section. It is entirely reasonable to be worried. After all, you are thrusting your cock through a hole. You don't know who or what is on the other side. Like a psycho who wants to damage someone's testicles. But let's be rational about this. Except for the at-home option, these Glory Holes are in public places. If someone assaulted you, you would likely be screaming in pain. In the process, the other guy might sustain injuries. Why would someone want to draw attention back to himself? Someone who despises gays might want to inflict violence. Then again, I couldn't imagine someone who hates gays feeling comfortable with an erection staring them in the face.

It is essential to have your phone handy, just in case something goes wrong. You may come across an individual who exhibits extreme behavior without any apparent cause. Do not interact with someone who is mentally unstable or angry; you will make things worse. Just walk away. So, while there is no reason to be irrationally fearful, use caution.

Meeting someone online is overwhelmingly safe. Most people you meet online are truthful and well-founded. The incidence of crimes stemming from these meetings is extremely low. Bottom line: use your judgment and be careful.

Legalities

The laws are different from state to state, even country to country. Therefore, it is advisable to use Google to research the legalities in your area. Here, I will discuss the topic in general terms. How legal are glory holes? Engaging in sexual activity in a public space is against the law. Lewd conduct, which is a misdemeanor, carries the possibility of arrest. That is a very low-class felony. But let's be rational about this. Should the police apprehend every individual engaging in sexual activity at a public place, it would lead to the collapse of the legal system. Do you have any idea how active these places are? Just like prostitution, it is widespread. The cops do not have the staffing to try and shut down every glory hole that exists.

I'm not saying there isn't a chance the cops will bust you. It might happen if the glory hole sex is taking place in an area accessible to the public, such as a restroom.

Outside public areas where glory holes are located, the police do not monitor private establishments like sex clubs or bathhouses. Because it's considered a private area. When you pay an admission fee upon entry, that venue is considered a private club. Sharing a booth with others is legal as long as the booth door remains closed. A closed booth door is akin to renting a hotel room.

Police only show interest in these establishments when they receive reports of drug use, dealing or trafficking. Other than that, the police are not concerned if two individuals engage in oral sex behind closed doors.

If you learn anything from this section, remember this. Do your homework on the law in your area and know your rights.

CHAPTER 5
Video or Bookstore

Both video and adult bookstores have back rooms where guys, regardless of their sexual orientation, can watch skin flicks in a private booth and play with themselves. Customers can also hop from booth to booth for one-on-one oral sex. Each location varies, with some booths arranged in a row. Other locations may arrange their booths in a maze to enhance the enjoyment of cruising. These booths host a diverse range of sexual activities. Since this book is about Glory Holes, I will focus solely on that aspect of sexual activity.

There are costs associated with entering the premises. In both places, you will have to pay an entrance fee. Some allow you to stay for as long as possible, while others have a time limit. Every place is different in terms of the number of hours you can stay.

In addition, the booths are not free. There is a general admission fee plus additional costs to rent a booth. These cubicles are for watching movies, which is the whole point of this setup. Some places require you to purchase tokens, allowing the user to sit in a booth and watch the movie. If you have tokens leftover, you can keep them for your next visit. Some places offer a user card instead of tokens. Like a debit credit card, you load it with cash. Other places don't provide the choice of a card or tokens, necessitating upfront cash payments.

These stores do not generate revenue from selling books or DVDs. Instead, the rental fees for a single booth occupancy provide the profits. Every place has a different setup. If you are looking for Glory Hole action, expect to drop a chunk of change into these booths to get your oral fix.

These Glory Holes are located on the adjoining walls between booths. Why is it not possible to access the holes from the outside, facing the hallways, for increased sexual activity? These stores aim to generate revenue. The profit lies in renting a booth for a movie. Having Glory Holes exposed to the open hallway is like giving it away for free. That is why Glory Holes are on the inside between rooms (to make money), rather than facing the outside (which loses money). These holes have a mini door, so you open or close the access on either side, depending on whether you are the giver or receiver.

Not all these stores will have individual video booths. Some stores may have one large, dark room at the back. An open concept will be on one side of the room, where you can watch videos and jack off. A confined area for sexual activities is located on the opposite side. There may be partitions with Glory Holes (again, between the adjoining partition walls). Whether in a booth or a dark room, the cruising etiquette is the same.

You have two options: either the giver or the receiver. You can sit and wait, or you can go cruise the halls. Waiting means you sit in a booth; door closed and wait for someone to come to you. Pull your pants down and stroke yourself, as watching porn will keep you erect and horny. Maintain focus on both the TV monitor and the Glory Hole. Pretty soon, you will find guys kneeling in front of the hole. Depending on what you want to do (give or receive), follow the etiquette rules I have described earlier. If the neighboring booth is only interested in watching a movie, you may have to leave and cruise.

Some places even have windows between the booths. The men on either side of the wall cannot see each other. Only when one of the men presses a button to reveal oneself can the other person see you. This signifies the individual's desire to view the other person through the closed window. The other person can do the same. Keep in mind that cruising for sex is entirely superficial. Rejection happens all the time. It's ironic since Glory Holes revolve around anonymous sucking. Despite this, men still desire to put a face on their dicks.

All of this reads harder than it sounds. To combat boredom, you spend plenty of time waiting, posing, leaning against the wall, and walking up and down the halls. You are eagerly anticipating the arrival of fresh meat. On the other hand, it's a buyer's market for those who are not picky. However, the reality is that gay men are selective. As a result, you must wait patiently, avoiding addicts and hustlers who are eager to sell their cocks for quick cash.

Some (but not all) bookstores and video sites exclusively cater to heterosexual men. Some straight men don't care if a gay guy sucks them off. To these men, a mouth is a mouth, no matter who is doing the sucking. But be careful. Not all straight guys are as liberated as you might think. You should conduct thorough research and familiarize yourself with the various straight video bookstores. Investigate hookup sites that feature discussion boards about these straight places. Read what others have to say about gay men cruising these straight Glory Holes. Ask as many questions as you can. You can also find websites that provide reviews and ratings for these types of places.

CHAPTER 6
Bars, Baths and Sex Clubs

Notwithstanding the video and bookstores, the only other Glory Holes in a safe and controlled environment are the baths and sex establishments. Backrooms in clubs and bars may also have Glory Holes, but their legality is determined by each jurisdiction.

Bars and Clubs

Because we are talking about gay men, businesses cannot stop two guys from hooking up on the premises. The cock wants what it wants. If management or security staff catch you, they may request your departure.

But not all bars or clubs are like this. Some places encourage guys to get sexually active, as it is beneficial for business. Some establishments have what is known as a dark room (or backroom). It is pitch-black in complete darkness. After a while, your eyes adjust, and you can make out shapes and figures. Guys will stand around and cruise, waiting for someone to come in. Alternatively, newly paired couples who met at the bar may enter the darkroom for a quickie, which features multiple booths. Couples primarily use these booths for privacy, as some prefer not to have an audience or worry about other men joining in. Thus, the booths allow couples to have their own space away from an audience. However, these booths incorporate an additional feature. They have Glory Holes in between or outside the booths. Each side has a door covering the hole, allowing the user on either side to open and close it at their convenience.

If you and your partner want sex, you can enter a booth and get busy. However, if you both decide to utilize the Glory Hole, you have the option to seduce each other through the opening. Alternatively, you could choose to use the same booth and open the small hole for some three-way action.

If your middle booth has holes on both ends, you can even attempt a four-way. Imagine each of you sucking off a cock. Or perhaps both of you want the experience of getting sucked off by two different men. The issue arises from the fact that you are unsure about the appearance of the anonymous man. Therefore, you must disregard caution and take risks.

If you find no one, you can wait in the booth until someone else starts to cruise. Just like all places to seek sex, there is always a significant amount of waiting. But when you hear someone enter the next booth, make your move and go for it. You have the option to either seduce the man or succumb to him.

The darkroom is not the only place where these glory holes exist. Gay bars and clubs often feature holes between their men's bathrooms. Because these establishments cater to the gay community, this is a better option than cruising a public bathroom. In a gay bathroom environment, it's highly unlikely that the police will bust you or that a patron will assault you. Gay men are aware that this is a common occurrence, which makes a gay setting feel much safer for them to cruise around in.

Bathhouses

Sex clubs and bathhouses operate in a similar manner. First, a little background. If you've read any of my writings, you're aware that I am the world's undisputed bathhouse expert (yes, I'm boasting, but it's okay to feel a little smug!). You can read a lot about the gay baths on my website, bathhouseblues.com.

Bathhouses are places for men to hook up for sex. They feature common areas and private rooms. Everyone strolls around unclothed, save for a waist-wrapped towel, which introduces the bath element. There are showers, saunas, steam rooms, and whirlpools to add to the wet bathhouse atmosphere. The baths offer a variety of features to keep guys engaged, such as the dark room, also known as a fetish room, which resembles the backroom of a club or bar.

All bathhouses rent private rooms to customers who want to have sex. Many of these rooms feature Glory Holes. Typically, these holes are located between the adjacent walls that separate the rooms. When you step into a private room, you might catch a glimpse of someone's mouth peering through a hole in the wall. But don't worry about having an audience. There are trap doors on either side of the hole. If you want privacy, you shut the door on your side. Some holes are even located on a room's door, facing right out into the bathhouse hallway. It is not unusual to be walking the halls of the baths and see a cock sticking out of the door of a room.

Sex Clubs or BDSM Dungeon

Gay sex clubs work a little differently. It functions similarly to the back room of a bar or club, but it encompasses the entire sex club! Bathhouses give the customers things to do during the down periods (sauna, steam, porn room). However, a sex club excludes these additional activities. It is narrower in its focus on the type of sex it promotes. It could be a jack-off club, where most guys sit around jerking off. It could be a porn lounge, where individuals watch a variety of gay skin flicks in separate rooms. It could be a club akin to a dungeon, equipped with slings and saddles, where individuals can engage in intimate activities.

Why do these sex clubs feature Glory Holes when sex is freely available? Cruising the toilets at a gay club is less risky than trolling for cock in a public washroom.

By playing out their fantasy in a bathhouse or sex club, men can act out in a safe and controlled environment under these conditions. Many couples visit the baths together to indulge in their fantasies and satisfy their sexual desires. Like the backroom of bars, these places also have dark rooms with booths for Glory Holes.

These places also feature a Slurp Ramp, with a row of ten to 20 Glory Holes positioned side by side. On one side, 10 to 15 guys stand in a row, sticking their cocks through each hole. On the other side, all these cocks are beside one another. One after the other. This allows men to perform multiple sucks consecutively, as all these cocks are beside one another. This allows men to perform multiple sucks consecutively. While this may seem thrilling to the recipient, it's important to remember that guys can be unpredictable. They need to attach a face to the cock or mouth. The guy sucking will often peek through the hole to see the other guy's face. If the guy is his type, he will suck. If not, he'll move on to the next cock. The same goes for the receiver. If the sucker is not performing satisfactorily, he will withdraw his cock and wait for the next individual. This approach undermines the essence of the Slurp Ramp's purpose—to suck every single cock blindly. That's men!

CHAPTER 7
Public Spaces

This book wouldn't be complete if we didn't talk about public sex—specifically, Glory Holes in public bathrooms.

This chapter only provides advice for **CONSENTING ADULTS ONLY**.

I **DO NOT** recommend trolling a public toilet for sex. There are just too many uncertainties. Seeking out sex in a gay environment is one thing. But, in my opinion, cruising for a blowjob in a heterosexual setting where anyone, especially those underage, walks in is too risky. The likelihood of a lewd conduct bust is exceptionally high. Look at George Michael. This could potentially land you on a list of sexual offenders.

Why do so many gay men love cruising for sex in toilets? For those men, public sex is the ultimate high. The thrill and excitement of potentially getting caught in the act makes the sex even more enjoyable.

Oddly, this seems to be the only way a closeted married man can get man-on-man action. The idea is that going to a gay environment is riskier than cruising for sex in a toilet stall!

Therefore, you must exercise extreme caution when soliciting sex in a public restroom. Finding a Glory Hole in a public bathroom is next to impossible. If a stall has a glory hole, maintenance will promptly replace the stall containing the hole. What straight man wants to use a toilet stall with a hole where the person next door can see you doing your business?

Therefore, searching for a Glory Hole in an office building, restaurant, or department store washroom is not feasible. The only places you might find Glory Holes are truck stops, gas station bathrooms, or public toilets located in parks. Many Glory Hole website directories will list these public bathrooms with Glory Holes in different states.

Any cameras in a bathroom are illegal, as they are considered an invasion of privacy. This explains why so much discreet sex occurs there. But a public bathroom does have a lot of traffic, with many comings and goings. Most guys go to the bathroom to take a leak or wash their hands, leaving the toilet stalls free for this activity. However, men do occasionally need to use the restroom to do the "number two."

While there are no cameras inside the bathroom, they exist both inside and outside the door. Many public washrooms unintentionally feature a warning signal when someone enters, such as a long entrance corridor or a noisy door opening. This helps avoid getting caught. It would also help if you had an escape plan ready. You never know what is going to happen. So, get to know those specific surroundings well.

When the public restroom is empty, inspect the layout. If multiple stalls are taken, leave and wait for the bathroom to be nearly deserted before entering a stall. Unlike women's restrooms, men don't hang out to chat. Most men's bathrooms are silent spaces. They come in, do their business, and leave. Therefore, take a seat in the stall that has a hole.

While sitting on the toilet, pay close attention to the traffic coming and going. After a while, you will be able to tell how many people come and go from the bathroom by ear. There will be times when you hear nothing but silence. There will also be moments when you hear a multitude of men entering and exiting.

Like any form of cruising, it involves a significant amount of waiting around. Therefore, you may have to wait for a considerable amount of time before any action occurs, as it is primarily a hit-or-miss situation. One suggestion would be to post an ad on a local hookup site stating that you are in this type of bathroom, waiting to give or receive in this stall. However, you expose yourself to the possibility of detection, or even worse, becoming the target of a gay basher.

Pay close attention when a guy sits on the toilet in the other booth. If he is taking a crap, don't bother trying to make a move. He's there for other business. However, if you hear nothing but silence, observe that his pants are around his ankles, and he is not taking a dump or a leak. Then you should proceed. The most non-threatening approach is to gently place your foot into the next stall. No reaction means no interest. If the other person's foot touches yours, you initiate the next move. If you want to give, lean in front of the hole and open your mouth. If you desire to receive, insert your cock into the hole.

Which actions should you take if someone enters while you're having fun? Quickly move back onto your toilet seat. Seeing two sets of legs facing each other between stalls would appear odd to the untrained eye. Once the person leaves, you can continue. Alternatively, you could simply decide to end the encounter and leave. It is your choice.

Be extremely careful, you never know who will walk through that door. It could be anyone, because this person is a stranger whose motives you don't know. Is he a psycho or a gay basher? Or is this a sting you've stepped into? The police and security are aware of these Glory Holes, and they closely monitor these public restrooms. But they cannot keep guard by the door 24/7. However, they do make random spot checks.

If the cops catch you having sex in a toilet stall, charges will depend on the arresting officer. Leaving the toilet stall door open during sex could increase the likelihood of charges, as it is legally considered an indecent act. Depending on how he sees the situation, the police officer will either let you go or charge you. If you refuse to provide your name or cooperate, the situation could worsen. All these factors could potentially persuade the officer to charge you with lewd conduct. Because this is a low-level misdemeanor, it all depends on the cop.

Regardless of what happens, keep the stall clean. Don't leave condoms on the floor or wipe cum on the stall door. This will only lead to complaints, prompting security to monitor the washroom area more frequently. Have fun but keep it clean.

Once again, I **DO NOT** recommend trolling a public toilet for sex. This chapter only provides advice for **CONSENTING ADULTS ONLY**.

CHAPTER 8
At Home Glory Hole

When combing through online ads, you will inevitably see ads for someone "hosting" Glory Hole action in their home. The typical ad would read something like this:

Seeking Discreet Glory Hole Action. Bi attractive 41 HWP 7.5 cut. Walk in through the unlocked door. Look for hardwood paneling to replace the door. Stick cock in and cum. Please be discreet. NSA.

The above ad is a perfect example of the Internet's ability for people to connect. Before the World Wide Web, there was no way to advertise Glory Hole action from the comfort of one's own home. Now it just requires clicking a switch, and you can send an ad to thousands in seconds. Millions can see these encounters on amateur gay porn sites and OnlyFans accounts. Why is it popular? The unknown thrill has sex more exciting for both parties.

The giver experiences excitement as they listen to their front door creak open, hear someone walking across the room, and witness a cock thrust through a hole. On the other side of the hole, the receiver has no idea what will happen once his erect cock enters the unknown, which makes it exciting for him.

However, this is not without its own set of challenges. Cruising for sex means endless game playing and waiting. However, this also applies to any form of online cruising.

Initiating a Glory Hole visit in someone's home is the same as arranging a hookup. The only difference is that you won't be having a face-to-face conversation with the host. The host will position themselves behind a wall, preventing you from seeing your trick.

When you arrive and open the door, you will immediately see the Glory Hole, which resembles a large piece of plywood with a hole in the middle. Drop your pants, insert your cock, and enjoy the blowjob. It is that simple.

For the person hosting (setting up the Glory Hole), you want to be 100% in control of the setting. Prepare for anything and everything by having a Plan B, Plan C, Plan D, and even a Plan E. You need to over prepare because anything could happen. I would strongly advise you to NOT do this at a location that is not yours, such as work or someone else's home. You lack control over the environment, which belongs to someone else. If your hookup results in damage to someone else's property, it is now your responsibility to bear the associated costs. In addition, you never know who is watching, as hidden cameras may lurk around.

I've already written about safety issues in "Where Can You Find a Glory Hole?". There are a few additional factors to consider. But making sure your hookup is a consenting adult is **your responsibility**. While only those who are 18 and older can post ads on gay online forums, it's important to note that people often lie. Therefore, it's advisable to limit your interactions to individuals who are similar in age. Later in this section, I will discuss the importance of screening processes as an additional layer of protection. If you are still paranoid about your safety, you can set up a discreet surveillance system. However, that violates the visitor's privacy, so I advise against it. If you feel your safety supersedes the other person's privacy, several spying options are available. Because I'm not familiar with them, I can't recommend any. However, you can research online. Even a Nanny Cam would work.

So how do you set up an at-home glory hole? Depending on your living situation, you have a few options.

If You Own A House

If you can access your basement door by descending a staircase into your cellar, that would be the perfect location for your at-home Glory Hole. It would give you the most privacy, as people outside can't see what's happening unless they walk on your property and watch from above. This locked door protects you and your belongings, as well as preventing intruders from entering your home. The door will have an opening that resembles a "pet door" (the entryway for pets to enter and exit the house). The only difference is the round hole and the elevated position of the "pet door" on the door itself. If you are making the hole yourself, make sure it is smooth and sanded. Guys don't want splinters on their cocks. As the host, you stand behind the locked door and wait for guys to show up. When the hole is not in use, keep it closed by installing a locked door from the inside. If you don't mind having a hole in your basement door, this is the best setting for an at-home Glory Hole.

The second-best way is to use your garage, but only if it has a door that leads into your house. Please refer to the previous paragraph on the basement door for instructions on how to create a glory hole on the entry door to your home. You should leave the large garage door wide open but position your car so that it obstructs the view of the door to your house. People won't be able to view what is happening because your car is camouflaging your activities. If your neighbors are nosy, they can only observe the number of men who visit your garage. However, it is important to keep your car locked and your vehicle's alarm system activated. Besides that, make sure there is nothing worth stealing in your garage. You might want to place one of those neighborhood cameras outside your garage, just in case. This does not constitute an invasion of privacy, as you are not recording the actual oral sex action. All you're doing is monitoring the guys coming and going from outside.

If a basement or garage door is not an option, your mudroom serves as an excellent alternative. The individual will access your mudroom through the front door. Its door separates the mudroom from the rest of the house. The sole distinction is the inclusion of a glory hole in the door. Again, please refer to the previous paragraph on the basement door for instructions on how to create a glory hole on the mudroom door.

For safety and security, update your home's door to one like that. If you can't afford a door or your house layout prevents it, get creative. You can put up some wall paneling, a removable door, or even a king-size mattress covering the entryway to your home from the mudroom. For the sucking to occur, all three options must have a hole or entryway.

Make sure your glory hole has a sturdy base. Please do not use a sheet or shower curtain, because the person on the other side will always put his weight against the glory hole. Using something as flimsy as a sheet will cause the person on the other side to collapse on you. This will lead to the complete disintegration of your at-home sanctuary.

Having a solid piece of wood with a hole in the middle is as simple as it sounds. Put a layer of covering around the inside of the hole. That way, the person on the other side doesn't get blisters. Additionally, if the individual is positioned behind the board, consider adding handles to support the person, as they will be pushed and pulled during the encounter. All of this depends on the Glory Hole remaining as sturdy as a rock (again, pardon the pun). It must withstand any chance of collapse. The last thing you want is a weak setup that can fall apart after the first hiccup. That is one way to kill the mood.

Finally, keep in mind all the different heights of men when making the hole. The hole itself should be wide enough for any guy to stick his cock through. But at the right height, any guy can use it without crouching or standing on their tippy toes. If none of these options work for you, consider setting it up in your backyard, provided that your fencing is high enough to prevent neighbors from seeing it. You have a self-standing door with a hole in it, and you wait behind it for your trick to come over. Sturdy chain-link fences could also be a viable option, as they feature holes at every height suitable for a man's cock. The only problem with this is that you have face-to-face contact, which somewhat defeats the purpose of an "anonymous" blow job.

If You Own An Apartment

You never want someone giving or receiving in the hallway outside your apartment door. Whether you like it or not, the person must enter your premises.

If you live in a condo, you probably will have a powder room near the front door area. Installing a glory hole in the bathroom door is a simple solution, allowing you to wait inside until the person arrives. As for the rest of the condo, look for an obstructionist device, such as a stair blocker, to send the message that the rest of your condo is off limits. However, you do run the risk of robbery, as you have allowed a stranger into your home. However, the same risk applies to any hookup you arrange. This is the chance all men take when inviting strangers over for sex. Make sure you leave instructions to shut the main door upon entering and exiting the premises.

If your apartment is a studio and the bathroom is located far from the central doorway, it becomes more of a challenge. The only option is to find wall paneling that will stretch to both ends of the walls in a hallway. When someone enters your premises, they will see a wall covering the entire entryway. Therefore, they are unable to proceed further. Finding something significant enough to block an entire hallway is a TALL order.

If there is no way to block access to the rest of your home and you want to remain anonymous during the encounter, setting up your Glory Hole in a hotel room is the last option. Renting rooms for hookups constitutes a lucrative portion of hotels' business. Plus, this is safer than inviting someone to your home.

But what if you encounter a maniac who wants to cut your cock off? You take the exact same risk when you arrange a hookup. Do you take any safety measures when you meet a random stranger for sex?

If so, then follow the same steps you used for that. If you don't have a plan, make one today. Before going, always email the hookup's handle and address to a friend. This ensures that if you disappear, there will be a record. The chances are slim that there is a crazy person behind that hole. But it can happen. The bottom line is to take the necessary precautions.

Items Needed

Put a "Welcome Mat" on the other side of the Glory Hole. The goal is not to greet your trick with a warm welcome. The goal is to prevent the spillage of multiple loads of cum on your hardwood floor. Instead, it finds its way onto the welcome mat. I wouldn't even bother to keep or clean the mat. I would discard it and purchase a new one the next time.

- Towels to clean yourself off.

- For any emergencies, have your cell phone handy and accessible. This is especially important if your trick turns out to be psychotic.

- Have a First Aid Kit handy, as you never know what will happen.

- For music, have Gay Porn playing in the background. It seems to make the encounter even hornier.

Chapter 9
Screening At Home

Some men don't discriminate based on the type of dick that shows up on their doorstep; they recognize that a cock is a cock. Which is something delicious to suck. But if you're like most gay men, the type of cock you'll blow is game-changing. Negotiating oral sex at home isn't different from the millions of hookups arranged online every second of the day worldwide. But since this is about Glory Hole sex, here are some tips to navigate your way to a successful blowjob.

Again, many men don't screen their blowjobs. In rare cases, you don't communicate with the person who placed the ad. It tells the person to go to a particular address, open the door, and get to business. This laissez-faire attitude is not a good idea unless the host doesn't care about potentially exposing their dirty laundry to the world.

If you are unconcerned with the individual's identity and are at ease sucking any erect penis, skip this section. However, like most gay men, you have your preferences. Cut or uncut? Big or small? Furry bush or shaved pubes? Be clear about your likes and dislikes. If you are not honest, you are wasting both parties' time. It is better to be upfront than neutral. In the long run, being truthful is better for both the giver and receiver.

Request a picture of their cock. Yes, we receive more cock photos than face pictures, but you need proof. People are dishonest, and descriptions may not accurately reflect what shows up. Again, this reduces the amount of wasted time. If you don't like what you see, you can move on. Additionally, men who have a picture ready to send you typically have more experience navigating through quickie sex situations like this. They can take direction, which means less drama and hassle.

If you clearly state what you like and dislike in your post, some guys may ignore it and contact you anyway. You can ignore their message or decline their offer. If they become angry, remain steadfast in your beliefs about what you are seeking. It is best to decline someone who is not your preference. If you don't, you're wasting both parties' time on an unpleasant encounter.

You receive a message from an individual; the cock image is satisfactory; what is the subsequent course of action? You send the person a set of instructions on what they should do. To enhance your safety, refrain from immediately disclosing your address to the person. You give him a "location" that you can see through your window. If you're staying in a motel, ask him to wait in the parking lot. If you're hosting from home, ask him to wait outside a specific house across the street. For condo or apartment hosts, find a place where he can wait outside your window. Some condos or apartments provide their residents with a live video of the lobby via their televisions or computers.

If men balk at these instructions, drop them. They are not worth it, which means they are trouble. This type of screening also allows you to make sure the person didn't lie. For example, a man may claim to weigh 150 pounds, but a 300-pound man may appear in the waiting area. That would allow you to quickly and easily dismiss anyone who is lying. You may see that someone followed the instructions, but something seems wrong. That's the beauty of this type of screening. You can cancel, and if he's upset, he can't find you. This is your hookup, and you're in charge. It's okay to cancel at the last minute. There is no need to offer any explanation to the other person. It is your decision, so don't feel guilty about changing your mind.

Conversely, you also experience no-shows in your role as host. You arrange everything; he sounds hot and sexy in your message exchanges, and you cannot wait to connect. Then nothing happens. He fails to show up, and your messages to him go unanswered. Many guys get cold feet. While conversing with you, they succumb to the lustful thrill. Once offline, they crash to earth. They begin to think rationally instead of impulsively, which can lead to feelings of fear. It's worse if they jack off after chatting with you. Because after ejaculation, once they have gotten off, all that horniness goes away.

If you are scheduling multiple blowjobs at your glory hole, it is vital that the guys who come over adhere to their time. If they don't stick to the schedule, many men will arrive within minutes. Warn your hookup that a late arrival might lead to cancellation. Otherwise, things could get backed up. Since you have arranged for them to wait in a designated area before coming over, canceling him if he is late, is no problem. Otherwise, rushing your session can lead to a less enjoyable experience for both of you.

If you are beginning the process of hosting "At Home" Glory Holes, schedule your blowjobs every 60 minutes. Consider scheduling three oral sessions in an afternoon, specifically at 1 PM, 2 PM, and 3 PM. Once you're comfortable, you can plan additional blowjobs, possibly every 30 minutes. Padding the appointments between blowjobs gives you time to rest and clean up.

Conclusion

Glory Holes truly represent what quick, anonymous, depersonalized sex is all about.

The whole concept of Glory Holes is to suck or get sucked, no matter what the guy looks like. It is important to remember that a cock is just that—a cock. However, men often exhibit superficiality, frequently seeking the appearance of their anonymous partner. So, keep that in mind when you start cruising Glory Holes for oral sex.

Special treat. Below are two true stories that have taken place at the gay baths. The first story recounts a person's experience at the Bathhouse Glory Hole. The second is about a married man obsessed with cocks. How does he handle it? You will have to read the story to find out.

My book, Gay Steam, features that story and many others. If you like it and want to read more steamy bathhouse stories, please go order your copy today at your favorite online retailer.

His Glory Hole Experience

During an out-of-town business trip, this bathhouse regular decided to drop by the local baths. This bathhouse has everything you can imagine. He was surprised to find his room equipped with a glory hole. For those of you who are new to the concept, a glory hole is a hole in the wall where a man can insert his cock. On the other side, someone else will perform oral sex. There is glory holes located on the premises of all bathhouses. Most likely, they will be in the dark areas of the baths.

If you are fascinated by Glory Holes but unsure where to look for them, the answer is simple: go to the gay baths. While you can find Glory Holes in a variety of locations, the gay baths are the safest place to experiment because of all the freewheeling sex that goes on. Bathhouses not only strategically place Glory Holes between rooms, but some even install them on the exterior walls. You can walk down a hallway and see a closed door, but you will also see a cock sticking out of a hole.

Bathhouses even have entire sections of their premises with nothing, but walls filled with Glory Holes. Some gay saunas construct vast Glory Hole play areas and set them up like a phone booth. You go in, stick your dick through a hole, and wait for someone to come by to suck you off. If you enjoy giving, wait for the cock and slurp. You have no idea who is on the other side, as it is dark.

The circular platform, however, is the centerpiece of this Bathhouse Glory Hole play area. Picture a vast circular tube with walls. Inside are holes where you can stick your dick through. Guys roam the outer perimeter, attempting to suck off as much as possible. If you seek anonymous oral action, this is the ideal place to be. Given the widespread presence of glory holes within a gay bathhouse, management probably tries to install them in every possible location!

What is the attraction to Glory Holes? Some guys want a quick blowjob, and it does not matter who does it. Most men are attracted to the idea of being anonymously blown, as are those who enjoy blowing anonymous dicks.

Most of these men enjoy oral sex, and the more cocks present, the better. They're not interested in talking, learning, or getting involved with the other person. They just want to suck cock, and they don't care who it is. In that sense, Glory Holes are excellent because they allow you to suck as much as you want.

On the flip side, for guys who can't get any action at the baths, Glory Holes fit the bill for a quickie. If they're not picky about who sucks them, it's a buyer's market. Glory Holes truly represent what quick, anonymous, depersonalized sex is all about.

However, not all men exhibit complete abandonment in their sexual behavior. Just as some men are selective about their hookups, the same applies to blowjobs. Men want to see the face that matches the cock. The out-of-state guy learned this fact at his first visit. The room he occupied had a glory hole that allowed him to see into the adjacent room.

There is a small door on either side, so the patron will have the option of closing his hole or leaving it open. Given his interest in voyeurism, he was excited by the prospect of witnessing some action from his vantage point next door. However, his excitement quickly turned to disappointment as no one showed any interest. Whenever he managed to secure a room with a glory hole during his subsequent visits, the man next door would notice him and promptly close it. The only ones who left their glory hole open were men over 65 or weighing 350 pounds.

However, there are instances when you can strike the right combination. One day, the out-of-state guy was given a room with a glory hole, and the guy next door left it open. The guy next door was blonde and skinny with a goatee. The guy from out of state undressed, put on his towel, and headed out for a shower. Before exiting, the out-of-state guy left his side of the glory hole open, just in case. When he got back, the out-of-state guy expected that the guy next door would shut their side of the glory hole. To the out-of-state guy's surprise, the other side was still open when he returned to his room. OK, the out-of-state guy thought. Perhaps the man next door enjoys having people witness his intimate moments. The out-of-state guy closed his room door (not the glory hole) and lay down on his bed to see what would happen next. The out-of-state guy heard some movement and got up to peer through the hole. The individual from out of state was able to observe the next-door guy, who was sitting on his bed, facing the hole, and stroking his cock. This individual from out of state followed suit, uncertain about the intended outcome.

Then the guy next door stuck his penis through the hole. The man from out of state froze, unsure of what to do, as he desired to receive rather than give. It's one thing to tell someone face-to-face that you don't suck cock. How can you communicate effectively when you have a dick stuck in your face through a hole? The only thing the out-of-state guy could do was stroke his cock. After a few minutes, the man next door withdrew his cock, prompting the out-of-state individual to insert his own dick through the opening. That is when the fireworks began.

The man next door began to devour the out-of-state individual as if he had not eaten in days. The out-of-state guy, his entire body pressed against the wall, was enjoying the blowjob. After 10 minutes, the individual from out of state withdrew his penis as he was on the brink of ejaculating. Then he caught a glimpse of the man next door, from his chin to his nose, as he adjusted his mouth and moved his lips and tongue, indicating his desire for more. The man from out of state offered him his balls, which the man from next door devoured. The hole was higher than his crotch, forcing him to stand awkwardly on the tips of his toes.

After five minutes, the out-of-state guy withdrew and asked the next-door guy what he liked to do. The next-door guy said he loved to suck dick. The out-of-state guy then asked if he could come over, and the next-door guy said sure. The out-of-state guy grabbed his key, left his room, and went next door. As the out-of-state guy lay on the bed, the next-door guy continued to suck him until he reached an orgasm, accompanied by screaming and exhaling.

The man from out of state rose from the bed, wiped himself off, kissed the man from next door, and expressed his gratitude for a wonderful time. The out-of-state guy then took another shower and thought, "Do I continue to leave my hole open or closed?" At that point, the out-of-state guy had only arrived 30 minutes ago. He still had five and a half hours left. Leaving it open would indicate he wanted more. Closing it would signal the end. The out-of-state guy is overly sensitive to other people's feelings, but only because he knows what rejection feels like. An appointment forced the out-of-state guy to leave an hour later, solving the problem. During that hour, the out-of-state guy cruised through the hallways, took a long hot dip in the whirlpool, and sat in the sauna. Upon returning to his room to prepare for his departure, he closed his Glory Hole door. When the out-of-state guy left, he passed the next-door guy's room and waved goodbye. The guy next door waved back.

You can understand why many men gravitate toward glory holes. If they are not going to get laid, getting blown off—even anonymously—is better than nothing. Given that the out-of-state individual is not receiving much attention (apart from this instance), it might be beneficial for him to hang out around Glory Holes. As I have said, it is better than nothing.

To read more stories from True Sex Tales From The Tubs, order your copy of Gay Steam at your favorite online retailer.

Hungry To Suck

His name is Martin. He is 40ish, rough-looking, with tattoos and long hair tied into a ponytail. Did I mention he is married and straight? So, what's he doing at the baths? Well, he loves cock. Let me rephrase that. He absolutely loves cock. However, he considers himself very straight. He has no attraction toward men. However, he has an insatiable appetite for sucking cocks. When he spots a dick hanging out, he exclaims, "Wowza!"

Martin is in a quandary because he loves women but not men. But when he sees an erect penis, you better get out of the way. He enjoys slurping someone's dick for hours on end. However, he doesn't like other guys touching him when performing oral sex. Martin will not kiss or touch any guy while sucking. All he wants to do is suck cock.

Martin is from a suburban blue-collar area and shares access to a computer with his wife. Paranoid about his wife monitoring his search history, he doesn't dare pursue local hookups online. But he did hear about the baths, and that is where he goes to get his fix. Martin considers himself straight, and going into a gay environment intimidates and scares him. However, the temptation and desire for an erect cock are too strong for him to ignore. Every time he goes to the baths, he must down a couple of liquor shots to get comfortable.

When I first saw Martin at 10 a.m., he was walking around naked, except for wearing a hooded jacket. He had been at the baths since 4 a.m., engaging in cock sucking all night long. Martin told me if there's a cock with a pulse, he will suck it. His record for cock sucking was in college. He spent an entire day—8 hours with a few breaks—sucking off his coach's cock.

Martin's favorite way to suck is for the recipient to repeatedly say the word "fag" while he slurps away. Afterwards, he enjoys cum shooting all over his face or inside his mouth. However, the thought of another guy touching him while sucking repulses Martin.

Martin loves his wife, but he can't give up on Cock. To satisfy his needs, he has asked his wife to consider a three-way relationship involving two men and himself. Unfortunately for Martin, his wife has consistently rejected the idea. However, he revealed to me that he had previously been in a four-way relationship, which involved two men and two women. Martin said having an MTF (male to female) fuck buddy would fulfill his dreams. His objective is to locate an individual who bears a striking resemblance to a woman, including breasts, yet still possesses a penis. Since he shares a computer with his wife, how could he connect with those types of trans people without his wife finding out his search history online? The only solution he found was to visit gay baths.

Martin feels compelled to visit the gay baths to satisfy his sexual cravings for cock. As time passed, Martin's behavior became increasingly strange. I saw him on a Saturday afternoon one weekend, which wasn't unusual. However, Martin's excessive drinking led him to become less diligent in concealing his double life. Martin told his wife he was going camping for the weekend. But in reality, he was spending the weekend at the baths. Martin struggled to handle the situation. First, his wife forced him to take the dog on his trip! His wife asked, "How can you go camping and not take the dog with you?" Since the gay baths do not allow pets, Martin had no choice but to lock his dog in his car. However, he intended to check on his dog about every four hours. Martin likely didn't want to spend the money on a kennel. Next, he planned to use his debit card to pay his bathhouse fee. Then, he promptly turned off his cell phone and proceeded to chase down every cock in the building while also taking shots of liquor every 15 minutes.

After 24 hours, his wife was frantic, unable to reach him. She investigated his debit card transactions online and discovered an unusual charge in the city. She believed he was in the woods. Has someone stolen her husband's debit cards? Did someone kidnap him, putting him in danger? Unaware of the bathhouse concept, she proceeded to contact the listed location for the debit charges. She asked if her husband was there and what the place was like. The bathhouse staff refused to say if her husband was there. However, they did inform her what type of place a bathhouse was. Panicked, she filed a missing person report. Meanwhile, Martin's level of intoxication rose with each cock he sucked.

I'm uncertain about the outcome of this scenario. All I know is that I still see Martin at the gay baths. No matter what story he told his wife, she must have bought it.

To read more stories from True Sex Tales From The Tubs, order your copy of Gay Steam at your favorite online retailer.

About Bathhouse Blues

Bathhouse Blues is the world-renowned expert on gay bathhouse etiquette and culture. He has been the author of his self-titled blog since 2001. It is still the only blog on the web to discuss bathhouse etiquette and culture. Numerous periodicals worldwide, including the Huffington Post and Unzipped Magazine, have referenced his bathhouse writings.

He is also a contributor to the website GayDemon.com and runs a second bathhouse site, BathhouseBlog.com.

Contact Bathhouse Blues

bathhouseblues.com

Twitter @bathhouseblues

DISCLAIMER

The material in this book is for adults only. The First Amendment of the United States of America Constitution and the Canadian Charter of Rights and Freedoms protect this book as a reference work for educational, informational, archival, entertainment, and other purposes.

This book offers no medical, legal, or related professional advice. We encourage the reader to apply the contained information with sound judgment and seek advice from a qualified professional when necessary. At best, the content provided in this book is of a general nature. The purpose of this book is to enhance, not replace, intimate relationships with another individual.

This text should not be considered advice for illegal activities. This text is for private consumption only. By using any of the material in this book, you agree that you know your local laws and accept 100% personal liability for any illegal actions you commit.

The author advocates absolutely no illegal activities of any kind and makes no express or implied warranties of merchantability, fitness for any purpose, or otherwise concerning this book, all references, and the information it contains. The author urges you to consult the appropriate licensed practitioner for medical, legal, or spiritual advice.

Neither the publisher nor the author shall be liable for any commercial damages, including but not limited to special, incidental, consequential, or other damages.

Before engaging in any sexual activity, be sure that you do not take risks beyond your level of experience, aptitude, and comfort.

Meeting someone online is overwhelmingly safe. Most people you meet online are truthful and well-founded.

Nothing is ever 100% safe. For your protection, always keep a record of where you are going and send the information to a friend. Never give your home phone number to a stranger. Always assume the person you are hooking up with is HIV positive.

Please do not take for granted that your partner will protect himself. It is your responsibility to play safely. People from all over the world are meeting in person and making their first contact online. These meetings result in very few violent crimes.

In the world of glory holes, poppers are the most common. Know beforehand how Amyl Nitrite might affect you both physically and mentally. In addition, research indicates mixing more than one party drug in the equation often leads to unsafe sex.

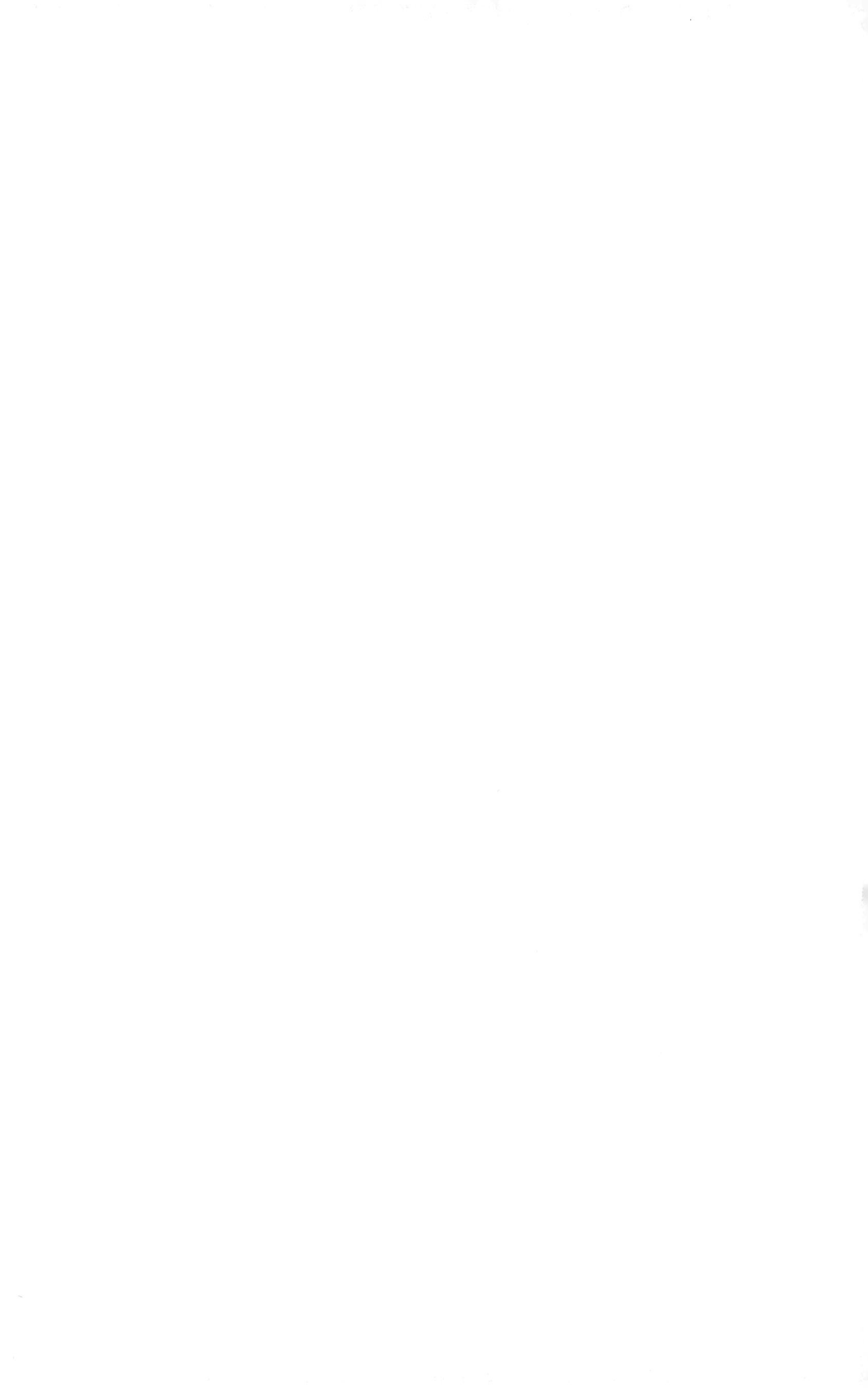